Praise for *A Husband's Guide to Hands-On Caregiving*

"Patrick Palmer has created an incredible book for all those who care for a loved one at home, especially male caregivers. Little or no resources have been available to guide these dedicated and loving supporters until now. This book describes ten critical segments of caregiving, all learned while on the job. These insights not only pertain to caring for a cancer patient but can be applied to those who care for someone with other debilitating diseases like ALS, dementia, Alzheimer's, stroke, etc. And it is not restricted to caring for a spouse. It also applies to caring for a child, parent, sibling, or friend. This is a must-read for those who are caregiving now or may be in the near future."

— Phyllis Levine, LICSW

A Husband's Guide to Hands-On Caregiving

Hard-Earned Lessons for Men—and Women—Caring for a Loved One at Home

PATRICK PALMER

ISBN: 1544264518
ISBN-13: 978-1544264516

To my loving wife, Angela, my hero, who battled cancer with strength and faith and never gave up.

.

CONTENTS

ACKNOWLEDGMENTS

With thanks to our children, Kirsten, Seann, David, and Sarah, whose love and support brought comfort to Angela and me.

Thanks to the incredible staff at Dana-Farber Cancer Institute in Boston, especially Dr. Patrick Wen, Dr. Eudocia Lee, and Sandra Ruland, R.N., who compassionately cared for Angela. Thanks also to Mary Bialer, owner of Snug at Home, and her team of Emma Friel, Catherine Farrell, Bridie O'Donnell, Yvonne Conway, Katie McCarthy, Katelyn McTavish, and Margaret O'Connell for their incredibly professional and loving care. To Peter J. Howe for his mentorship and huge support during the writing of this book. And to Marie B. Morris for editing and literary guidance.

INTRODUCTION

THE MOMENT the neurosurgeon told us that my wife had been diagnosed with Stage IV brain cancer, my world came crashing down. It was September 2011, and the prognosis was that she had six to twelve months to live. We had maybe one more year together? This was the most horrific news that I had ever been given. How was I going to care for her, and who was going to show me the way? I had to learn how to be a caregiver on my own. In this book, I want to share with you the many challenges I faced and how I overcame them, in the hope that I may be able to help you if and when you become a caregiver.

My partner, wife, and best friend, Angela Zambon Palmer, a 10-year breast cancer survivor, died on February 15, 2016, from glioblastoma multiforme. She was sixty-eight years old. She had lived for fifty-three months after that day in the doctor's office, far beyond her original prognosis. And for that four and a half years, I dedicated myself to providing Angela with the most loving and committed care possible.

AARP estimates that there are roughly forty million caregivers in this country. These are people caring for a spouse, parent, child, other family member, or friend. Approximately forty percent, or sixteen million, are men.

Caregiving by men can present a different set of challenges compared to women, who are naturally more nurturing. In 2001, when Angela was diagnosed with breast cancer, I learned about caregiving on the go. On my own, I had to rethink how to do basic things. No one was there to tell me how I was going to feel or how to cook dinner. When I needed it—in 2001 and again in 2011—information about what to expect, emotionally as well as practically, was surprisingly hard to find. To my knowledge, hospitals and cancer institutes offer minimal resources specifically for male caregivers.

My opinion is that you cannot counsel someone about caregiving unless you have been a caregiver yourself. In this book, I talk about what I learned from the hard knocks of hands-on caregiving. There is very little information out there for male caregivers, so I have made it my quest to share this knowledge. It is a "here's what I learned" discussion based on six years of caring for my wife.

This information is not specific to caring for someone with cancer. And it's not just for spouses. It is really for anyone who is taking care of someone who means a lot to him (or her): child, spouse, parent, sibling, close friend. And it can include a wide array of diagnoses: cancer, Alzheimer's, ALS, stroke, paralysis, or any other debilitating condition. Because there are minimal resources about caregiving by men, my target audience is mainly men—but many women may take away valuable insight and suggestions from my story.

Everything I talk about may not apply to you in the same way that it did to me. But there are bound to be common threads, especially when it comes to emotions. I am not presuming to be a therapist or social worker. What I will talk about is what I experienced.

LESSON 1

ALLOW YOURSELF TO BE ANGRY AND DEPRESSED

I WAS MAD AT GOD. Why Angela? Why me? What did we do to deserve this? Angela's lifestyle was impeccable. We were happy. We embraced life. We had four wonderful children, were professionally successful, and regularly donated to various charities. We believed in God and always lived our lives with the attitude that we were inferior to a more powerful being. We were good Christians. And I certainly had no anger toward Angela. This wasn't her fault. But I was angry about the fact that our life together was cut short. We were always talking about the future, whether it was traveling the world, buying a winter place in the South, or never retiring.

Over time, my anger has diminished, and I have acknowledged the fact that we were not the only ones who were facing death. Thousands of people are experiencing this every day. I didn't like it, but I started to accept it. It's a natural transition. This process may take longer for some than for others.

Depression is a very natural emotion to experience. I have self-diagnosed myself with seasonal depression. The older I get, the less tolerant I am of winter weather. Combine this with the knowledge that my wife was terminally ill, and I had times when I was incredibly low. I spent many a night crying myself to sleep.

When you love someone as much as I loved Angela, one natural reaction to a diagnosis like hers is to bargain. I prayed to God to have me trade positions with her; I wanted to take the bullet for her. I wanted to do anything I could to reverse direction. It was a horrible feeling to think that I couldn't do anything about her situation. This also fed my depression.

Throughout the course of her illness, especially during the last two years, I was no longer working. This transition, after forty-four years of employment, was especially challenging for me. My "new normal" routines were of a caregiving nature only. My objective was clear: to protect and care for Angela. But this limited my thinking and my personal aspirations. All of a sudden, I did not have anything to look forward to. I knew Angela was on a limited timetable and that we would not be able to realize our dreams.

I refused to become dependent on sleep aids to ease my depression. My doctor prescribed just six pills, which were helpful for the first two weeks after Angela's death. But I knew that I could become emotionally dependent on them, which would not be a good thing. Aware of the opioid and heroin addictions that are rampant in our society today, I knew that I did not want to head down that road.

I believe there is no short-term fix for

depression. My way of dealing with it is to be distracted. That means spending time with family and friends, playing golf, working out, journaling, and going to our home in Maine. Apart from writing this book, I try not to be reclusive. For me, being alone breeds depression.

Certain triggers and stimuli set off moments of depression. They could include seeing your loved one's clothes in the closet, catching sight of photos around the house, or even the delivery of mail addressed to that person. I am not suggesting that you remove all of your shared memories. For some, like me, clearing away everything that reminds me of Angela would be more depressing. I have removed her clothes from our closet, but they are in the cupboards in other bedrooms and in containers in our walk-up attic. In that way, I can choose to remember happy moments I associate with what she wore.

I also have all the photos of her and us in the same locations they were in before her death. Yes, at times, they can evoke great memories, but they can also bring me down when I think that I will never be able to enjoy new experiences with her. I have accepted that she has died, but that acceptance does not obliterate depression. Someday, I hope it does.

About two years before Angela's death, I reached out to the staff at her hospital, Dana-Farber Cancer Institute, and asked for a referral for a therapist in Newton. She is Phyllis Levine, a wonderful social worker. What attracted me to her was the fact that she had cared for her husband at home through terminal pancreatic cancer. Her daughter was later diagnosed with Hodgkin's lymphoma, and Phyllis herself is in remission from gastric cancer. She understands the world of cancer and caregiving and the emotions that go along with it.

Phyllis spent many hours with me, and I slowly began to understand my emotions: shock, fear, guilt, anger, and depression. What I was feeling was very normal for my situation. I began to accept the fact that these emotions would come and go and that I shouldn't fight them. Once I accepted this, my life became more manageable. And so can yours. Finding the right therapist will go a long way toward helping you understand and deal with your emotions.

The vast majority of hospitals have social workers on staff. When you seek out this sort of help, the success of the match depends on what you're looking for. If your concerns are related to the emotions of caregiving, you may have a tough time finding someone who has had that specific experience. On the other hand, if the issues you hope to work through are more general in nature, a good social worker can be very beneficial.

LESSON 2

ACCEPT HELP FROM FAMILY AND FRIENDS

WE HAVE BEEN TRULY BLESSED with a loving family and very supportive friends. We were fortunate that three of our four children live close by and our fourth is a one-hour flight away. They came by the house often and spent quality time with us, time I know Angela cherished. Other family members were frequent guests at the house, which really lifted all our spirits.

Friends that Angela and I made over the thirty-five years we spent together always kept in touch with us, and they made many trips to see Angela and offer support to me and the kids. Those are the best type of friends: the ones who are with you in good times as well as bad. But you may have to decide which ones are really there for you and which ones have become emotional burdens. Some friends turned out to be high-maintenance, and their visits would drag me down. I know their hearts were in the right place, but when you are emotionally stressed, taking care of someone else's issues can be too much. It became necessary to diplomatically tell these few friends that I needed to focus more on my family and less on others.

When Angela came home from her two surgeries, I assumed that I could take care of her myself. What I didn't contemplate was all the other things that I had to do.

For the first two years, I was handling things pretty well. But then I started getting overwhelmed. It was suggested to me that I should secure the services of a caregiver. I arranged to have someone work during the day while I was at the office. Soon afterward, I took a leave of absence from work so I could spend as much time as possible with Angela. I severed ties with the caregiver, but I quickly learned that that was a mistake.

Without my realizing it, my stress levels were rising. I was doing virtually everything myself. Not only was I grocery shopping and cooking meals, but I needed to keep the house clean. I was doing all the laundry as well. What's the big deal? People do this all the time. But throw into the mix the need to care for my terminally ill wife, and I was overloaded.

By not being shy in asking for help, I was able to do things that I hadn't done much for a couple of years. Friends were calling with tee times at my golf club, which allowed me to focus on something other than my caregiving requirements. In addition, I would retreat to our home in Maine for a couple of days every three weeks or so, allowing me to enjoy recreational activities like boating and fishing. Even in the winter months, I would enjoy those two-day breaks.

Enlisting the help of family members to stockpile meals really helped when I was alone at home with

Angela. When the inventory of meals became depleted, I hired a woman to prepare five dinners a week, delivered on Mondays. This worked very well for about three months, until she died unexpectedly. I now needed to reach out to others for help in this area. Again, visiting family members became engaged in cooking meals and shopping for us. They also taught me how to make nutritious meals and stay within a budget. This helped a lot, because I was not a smart shopper. I never compared prices and I always "overshopped." They taught me what to look for and what to avoid. This proved to be very useful when Angela died and I was shopping for myself alone. Meal planning and preparation for one can be a huge challenge. I threw out a lot of food initially, but I continue to learn from others how to plan and to accept the fact that leftovers are not a bad thing.

Some guys may be hesitant to ask for help. Men, the "fixers" in life, all too often feel that they can handle anything. Their egos can also prevent them from reaching out for help, like asking for directions. I was the same way. But there comes a time when you recognize your own frailty. There are many times when you can handle everything, but not when you are caregiving. Your emotions get in the way, and you realize that you can't fix everything all the time. It's hard to face that reality. It may be helpful to view the situation not with a sense of failure but by recognizing that asking for help is a sign of strength. Being able to recognize your shortcomings and do something about them goes a long way toward lifting the burden of bearing the total responsibility yourself.

I became adept at asking for help. Once I understood my limitations, physically and emotionally, accepting offers of help and directly asking for assistance became easier. I didn't hesitate to ask my kids to help me when the boats in Maine had to be winterized and stored and the outdoor furniture needed to be put away—not only up north, but at our home in Newton as well.

Caregiving is a full-time job. You need to reduce the stress of doing everything yourself by enlisting those around you to help out. Friends and relatives may volunteer, but sometimes they won't (perhaps because you've rejected their offers of help in the past). Don't be shy in reaching out for assistance.

During Angela's ordeal, our children and their spouses were tremendously helpful with caregiving. In addition, their love and support were a true inspiration to the two of us. They were facing challenges, too. They were also grieving, knowing their mother would not be with us for too much longer. They had children and jobs, so they were able to get mentally and physically away from the grim reality of what was happening. But the emotional strain was always present. We were all in this together, and we needed to be crutches for one another.

LESSON 3

CONSIDER HIRING HELP

IN JUNE 2013, Angela suffered a mini-stroke. Eight months later, she had another stroke and a seizure. After a few days in the hospital, she was dispatched to a rehabilitation facility to recover. Over the next three weeks, Angela had daily physio and occupational therapies. When she plateaued in her therapies, it was time for her to be discharged, with the strong recommendation that 24/7 caregivers be in the house. Although she could walk with assistance, it was obvious to all of us that she couldn't be left alone. Angela was a very determined person, and falling was a major risk. I was determined that she would not spend whatever time she had left in an institution.

The head nurse recommended a caregiver to me, and we immediately got together. After I asked around about her and her company, we entered into an agreement. She put together a group of professional caregivers. I was also a member of the team. Now I was able to relax a bit knowing that someone, whether it was me or one of the other caregivers, would always have Angela in sight. And this was not a one-person job. Having at least two people around the majority of the time bolstered Angela's safety. Although she was fairly mobile, she was also a fall risk, and she had a history of seizures and mini-strokes. Having more than one caregiver on-site enhanced her care and gave me peace of mind.

As in all relationships, not everyone is going to be a good fit. If and when you hire a private caregiving company, everyone involved must understand that you, as the primary caregiver, will be part of the decision-making process at all times. Even though all of our caregivers were certified, no one knew my wife better than I did. Angela was also part of the process until her health declined to the point where she could no longer contribute. When I was in the house, I would make the final decision regarding what a caregiver wished to do with Angela, whether moving her from the bed to the recliner, taking her downstairs for a meal, or performing range-of-motion exercises. Many functions did not need my input, such as dressing her, performing tasks to make her feel better like doing her nails, or taking her vitals.

Because I hired help, the company owner worked for me, and by extension, the other caregivers worked for me as well. The owner handled the administrative functions of running her company and scheduling her employees. Whenever we needed to add a new caregiver, my approval was always requested. And not all of the company's, or my, choices worked out. That's just part of the process. There will always be a certain level of turnover. The one constant is that your loved one is the focal point of whatever arrangement you make, and that his or her care is of the utmost importance.

LESSON 4

TAKE CARE OF YOURSELF

WHEN ANGELA was released from rehab, I developed some health problems of my own. I was having digestive challenges, including acid reflux and several loose stools on a daily basis. Our primary care physician referred me to the gastroenterology department at Brigham and Women's Hospital. I underwent a colonoscopy and endoscopy, and had fecal, blood, and lactose-intolerance tests. I had also experienced allergies for the first time. I was tested by an immunologist who noticed sensitivities to grass, tree molds, shellfish, and other allergens. He said people can develop them at any age.

The long and short of it, according to my gastroenterologist, is that these symptoms were most likely triggered by the stress I was under. Emotional stress can manifest itself in physical challenges. Over my lifetime, I have seen people develop panic attacks, acid reflux, chronic headaches, extreme anxiety, loss of appetite, high blood pressure, and a multitude of other ailments.

It can be difficult to recognize the stress you may

be under. The fact that Angela was receiving 24/7 care, that I was officially retired, and that I needed to find the resources to afford our new lifestyle meant that I was under severe stress without really knowing it. Family and friends would tell me that they noticed my weight loss, hyperactivity, inconsistent sleep patterns, and questionable diet. I realized that I needed to do something about it.

I was always an active person, especially when I was working at the Y. It was a busy job in which I oversaw major renovations to the facilities on top of day-to-day operations and community relations. Starting when I took a leave of absence, and more so when I took early retirement to care for Angela, my physical activity dramatically decreased even though I was a full-time caregiver. Without work to distract me, I became more absorbed in my own fear of what was going to happen. I felt incredibly sorry for Angela, but I also became a victim of my own sorrow. I needed to become more active.

Over the six years of caregiving, many people said that I needed to take care of myself in order to provide the optimum level of care for Angela. I would react to that by saying, "Yeah, yeah, yeah, whatever." That was my stubbornness kicking in. I kept putting that advice on the shelf until I realized that it was more than just a truism.

I joined Boston Sports Clubs, which had a location about one mile from the house. I developed a regular workout routine including strength, cardio, and stretching regimens. Over the next few months, I noticed a remarkable increase in my strength, energy, and overall wellbeing. I spent less time feeling sorry for myself and more time focusing on the job at hand. Caregiving for Angela was not a one-person operation. All of us had to be in the game all the time. Taking care of myself helped me take care of her.

What I did not expect was the physical fallout I experienced after her death. Once the shock wore off, I noticed extensive pain in my rotator cuffs and right hip flexor. These conditions grew out of over 2,500 transfers of Angela in a lifting and turning operation. This was not a one-man show. Over time, it became clear that we needed a minimum of two caregivers for any transfer, so I needed to be there. It was practically and financially impossible for our caregiving company to staff more than one person per twelve-hour shift.

At the time, you rarely think about the pain, but when it was all over, the reality of it hit home. My doctor prescribed physical therapy, and I am still a patient. I know that my insurance will eventually cut me off, so I have developed a large inventory of exercises that I will employ in the future. In addition, I enlisted the leadership of a personal trainer who puts me through supportive routines to complement the PT.

Phyllis, our social worker, was integral in helping me deal with my emotions during the last two years of Angela's life. You can't do it alone. It took me quite a while to understand that. Once I figured that out, and after several meetings with her, my emotional health improved.

I also derived stress relief by going regularly to our

home in Maine. It was a place that Angela and I loved, where I could be totally alone to fully absorb the pleasures of nature. Especially in the summertime, I could be outside for hours, whether fishing off the dock, taking care of the flowerbeds, or reading while reclined in a lounger. Being alone allowed me to remember the happy times with Angela at the lake house without experiencing sadness. It was a positive form of therapy.

If I had not done the things I did, I believe that my health would have nosedived. I needed to be there for Angela. And the only way that was going to happen was to take care of myself so that I could take care of her. I knew my responsibility was to be there. If I became ill and was unable to take part in caregiving, I can only imagine the strain and potential physical harm that the other caregivers could be subjected to in the long term. I sucked it up and got my act together.

Even after your loved one has passed on, continuing to take care of yourself is paramount. I have found it necessary to have physical therapy and two training sessions weekly. In addition, I have learned to eat a balanced diet. It is all too easy to rely on fast food and soda. You should consult with your doctor about seeing a nutritionist. Most practices have at least one on staff. I now have a vast amount of literature to read and learn from. And don't forget your therapist or social worker. I continue to see mine every three weeks. Taking care of yourself is not just limited to your body; you need to heal emotionally and mentally as well.

LESSON 5

EQUIP YOUR HOME

DURING the last two years of Angela's life, it was obvious that both of our houses needed changes to maximize her safety. Although she could walk with assistance initially, it was clear to all of us that stair climbing was becoming more of a challenge. I researched various suppliers of "stair chairs" and settled on one that had a leasing alternative. They are quite expensive to buy, and I wouldn't recommend purchasing one unless it will be in place for several years. In our case, we knew it would be used for several months, not years, which made a monthly rental far more practical.

I placed a wheelchair at the top of the stairs and one at the bottom. Angela was able to operate a chair but needed assistance to get in and out. In Maine, she was able to walk up and down stairs with a caregiver at first. However, in the eighteen months before her death, she was unable to walk with any stability. At that point, I converted the den on the first floor into a bedroom for her so there was no need for her to negotiate the stairs. In addition, a gait belt helped all of us to ensure her stability when she was standing.

As time went on, Angela became less able to get on and off the toilet. It was necessary to pull down her pants and pull them up when she was in a standing position. I installed grab bars in front of the commodes so that she could stabilize herself while one of us positioned her pants. This soon became a two-caregiver operation—one to ensure that Angela was balanced, and one to handle the pants.

Bathing also became a challenge. I equipped the walk-in shower with grab bars as well. As her illness progressed, it became very hard for Angela to remain standing while being washed. A shower chair allowed her to be bathed in a sitting position. This was easier on her but did require more than one caregiver. One or both of us would be soaked, but a shower was very soothing for her.

In the last year of Angela's life, walking became too strenuous for her. As a result, in order to take her out of the house, we needed to use a wheelchair to get her to the car. I contacted the stair chair supplier and rented a portable ramp that could be stored at the side of the house. This was the only way we could negotiate the three steps at the entrance.

Approximately four months before Angela's death, when positioning her in our king-sized bed was becoming unmanageable, the owner of our caregiving company recommended moving a hospital bed into the master bedroom. It was adjustable and on wheels, which allowed us caregivers to attend to her needs from both sides of the bed. The ability to raise her head and legs made it more comfortable for her, especially when she wanted to watch TV. When she declined further, we needed a Hoyer Lift, a hydraulic device that allowed us to mechanically raise her from the bed and place her onto a recliner in the bedroom. By this point, Angela was incontinent, so transfers to and from the bathroom were unnecessary.

When Angela returned from rehab, our oncologist sent a prescription to the Visiting Nurse Association. After an initial visit from a nurse, Angela was able to receive occupational and physical therapies at home at no cost to us. As time went on and she needed various types of equipment, these were also supplied free of charge. They included a wheelchair, walker, grab bars, hospital bed, supplemental oxygen, and Hoyer Lift. By contacting our local senior center, we were able to borrow a second wheelchair for as long as we needed it. In addition, when she entered hospice care at the house, a registered nurse visited weekly and supplied us with Angela's medications, again at no cost.

LESSON 6

DEEPEN YOUR FAITH

REGARDLESS of your religious persuasion, there is a "God" in your life. Even if you do not have a named religion, there must be someone or something that you believe is a supreme being through whom you live your life. And when you become involved in a situation like caring for a terminally ill loved one, it's OK to question and even to become angry with that God.

When Angela was diagnosed with brain cancer, after having gotten over the shock, I became mad. Initially, I wasn't sure with whom I was angry. From a selfish point of view, I was upset with Angela for disrupting our future plans and knowing that the life we had was now over. And then I thought, how could I possibly be mad at Angela? She's the one who became ill through no fault of her own. That anger was replaced with guilt for even thinking that way. I was still mad, though. But at whom? I concluded that it was God.

I knew that I needed to resolve this issue with God. Faith is very personal. I was hurting but didn't want to lose my commitment. I grew up as an Anglican and spent my teen years as an acolyte in our church. I served my priest probably four days a week. Five friends and I were deeply committed to our religion. As time went on and we all relocated to various new cities, the formality of my faith began to decline. I then met Angela, who was a devout Catholic, and I became religiously engaged once again. Our lives became well balanced.

I knew that I wanted to find this stability again. It wasn't just a matter of regular church attendance but more of a need to have conversations with God. I did that a lot. It happened at any time during the day, not just at home or in church. I felt the best time for this was when I was in the car alone. It wasn't necessarily a silent conversation but one that could become quite heated at times. I was mad and frustrated, but verbalizing my emotions helped. Over time, even after my anger subsided, I was still hurting. I offered up my pain to God.

By doing this, I noticed a relief of sorts in knowing that someone else was helping me through the discomfort. Having faith in God and believing that help is always available through prayer can be an amazing experience. It's not just sloughing off your hurt onto someone else, but sharing it. In much the same way that you seek help from family and friends, this is another source of help.

After five years struggling with coming to terms with God, I have more peace now. Reaffirming your commitment to Him is not an overnight process. It's a lifetime effort, and I am sure that I will be challenged again sometime in the future. But I am glad that I put in the effort. I would be very regretful if I just gave up on my faith.

Being in this comfort zone with God will help with the grieving process. As much as you may rely on a therapist or bereavement group to help you move on, faith also plays a major role. I have found that once my anger subsided, my belief in God increased. I rely on prayer to help satisfy a lot of anxieties that come my way. And I feel fortunate to have reaffirmed my belief. It will continue to be a blessing for the rest of my life.

LESSON 7

BE FINANCIALLY PREPARED

WE HAD GONE to a financial planner to map out our retirement. One of the recommendations was to obtain a long-term care insurance plan, which we did. That plan helped with Angela's at-home care.

Having 24/7 caregivers in the house comes with a significant cost, but it was well worth it for Angela's comfort and safety. The cost of this care was more than $430,000 for the final two years alone. Anticipating the cost, I collapsed a 403(b) and had Angela's pension cashed out. However, that was not going to cover our total living expenses. I was receiving only my two pensions, and we had a house in Newton and a home in Maine to pay for.

Our long-term care policy had a total value of over $600,000 but a maximum monthly benefit of approximately $8,000. Before we needed 24/7 caregivers at home, the plan covered certain other expenses. We had short-term caregiving for eight hours a day, which was covered. In addition, snow removal, landscaping, and housecleaning were paid for. When Angela required full-time care, it cost

$18,000 a month, of which around $8,000 per month was reimbursed. All in all, the plan paid close to $300,000. In addition, medical expenses not covered by a long-term care policy are tax-deductible.

I felt at some point that we could run out of money. I even considered that I might have to sell our Newton home or take out a line of credit against the significant equity we had in the house. But I could not conceive of moving Angela into another house. It would have been too hard on her physically and emotionally. And then I discovered that Angela's life insurance policy from her university had an accelerated death benefit. This provision allowed me to receive fifty percent of the value of the policy as long as her doctor felt that she had less than six months to live. Her doctor completed the necessary paperwork, and I was now confident that we had sufficient funds to cover all our expenses.

Everyone's financial situation is different. We were fortunate to have the resources that we did. If we had not, her care would have been far different. In hindsight, buying that long-term care plan was a great move. But remember, the older you are when you take out the policy, the more expensive it will be. In my opinion, it was still a great investment. Without it, we would not have made it financially.

Many people are under the mistaken impression that when someone becomes ill, health insurance will pay for all required care. That is simply not the case. Policies vary regarding how much is covered and for how long. When Angela was in rehab, our policy did not cover the total time she was there, and we paid out of pocket for about one week's worth of care. When we transitioned to Medicare with a supplementary plan, we had an easier time. As I mentioned, I was determined to care for her at home. If I had wished to transfer her to a rehab facility, Medicare would have covered a limited amount of time. After that, I was responsible for her care.

It is unfortunate that insurance plans do not cover private care at home. It has been proven that people who are cared for in their own home have a longer life expectancy. However, everyone may not be able to give the care at home that is required. Caregiving is very stressful and expensive.

If you decide to care for your loved one at home, you must understand that it can be a considerable financial commitment depending on the amount of time that caregiving is required. If you don't have a long-term care insurance plan, other sources of money must be found. First, determine how much equity you have in your home, and consult a loan officer at your bank to determine how much cash can be made available through an equity line of credit. If this is not a viable option, determine how much the bank will lend you. Second, you may have to sell stocks or bonds. Third, you may have to approach family members and ask for help.

Full-time caregiving in the home will cost approximately $25 per hour, or $600 per day. Depending on how long you require this care, you may be able to reduce your cost by fifty percent if you have someone in the house for only twelve hours. As I've mentioned, initially we needed eight hours per day of care. However, when Angela was released from rehab, we needed round-the-clock care due to her fall risk. In time, her mobility decreased, and I needed to assist whoever was in the house when it became impossible for one caregiver to provide all that was needed.

Everyone's case must be analyzed to determine the amount of care that is required. If your loved one suffers from a mental condition but is physically able to get around the house and perform personal functions like using the bathroom and showering, the level of caregiving may be less than what is required for someone who is physically challenged. Your financial obligations will vary along with your loved one's needs.

LESSON 8

BE READY FOR THE END

ANGELA NEVER gave up on anything, and when she was diagnosed with brain cancer, she was determined to beat it as she had beaten breast cancer. She became her own cheerleader, and her attitude helped me more than I can say. I revered her strength. As the months passed, the cancer took its toll, and in January 2016, Angela entered hospice care.

When it becomes apparent that your loved one's life is limited, you can help with the final transition in several ways. The initial step is to set up hospice care in the home or, if the patient is in a facility, ask the staff to do so. If the patient is at home, the treating doctor can order hospice care through the Visiting Nurse Association. In either case, the person holding the health care proxy signs a do-not-resuscitate order, or DNR. In essence, this means that the patient will not be placed on life support should he or she suffer a life-threatening event such as a stroke or heart attack. However, if the patient falls and breaks a bone, that would be treated. In addition, while in hospice, the patient will receive regular visits from a registered nurse, and all medication and supplies will be provided at no cost to the family.

To make the transition from life to death less overwhelming, efforts should be made to organize the patient's estate. Locate his or her will, insurance policies, bank and credit cards, pension information, IRA statements, information regarding funeral arrangements, and any special bequests. In addition, you should be in contact with an attorney who specializes in estate planning. Without knowing it, you will be in shock at the time of death even though it was expected. You can be prepared for the end, but you're never ready for it.

You should also put together a phone list of those you want to contact at the time of death. This list can be divided up among other family members so that you don't have to make all the calls yourself. The key calls that you have to make are to your immediate family. In our case, I was the last to know: the caregiver on duty made the calls to our two daughters and one son. The other son was in the house, and he was the one who woke me and told me of Angela's death. As a matter of fact, he waited until the other children arrived at the house so we could all say goodbye together.

The caregiver also made the appropriate calls to the Visiting Nurse Association and the funeral home. The registered nurse on call is the one who officially confirms the patient's death, so there is no need to call for an ambulance and have him or her transported to a hospital to declare the patient's death. In addition, our caregiver called the funeral home.

Once her body was removed from our home, everyone went home and tried to sleep. I had arranged through the caregiver to have all medical support items removed from the house the very next day, as I wanted to begin the grieving process. By the end of the day, our bedroom and the whole house looked the way they had before Angela's diagnosis.

LESSON 9

REIMAGINE SPECIAL DAYS

IT HAS BEEN almost a year since Angela's death. There were many milestones to get through. The first was my birthday, which fell on the day after her death. Angela had always gone out of her way make my birthday a very special day. Fortunately, our children filled that void, and we were able honor my day a couple of weeks later.

Other critical occasions followed: her birthday in May, Mother's Day, our anniversary in August, Thanksgiving, and finally Christmas, her favorite holiday. Initially, I had no interest in getting a tree, putting up outdoor lights, or decorating the house the way she had. Again, our kids came to my emotional rescue, and we all shared in the holiday rituals. Instead of Angela and me decorating the tree, our grandkids pitched in and created a lasting memory. But one hurdle remained: what to do on the day itself?

After a lot of discussion, we all concluded we would celebrate Christmas at our house. After our kids spent the morning opening presents with their kids, all eighteen members of the family attended church together and convened at home. The remaining gifts were distributed, and we were ready to break bread together. Everyone pitched in by bringing various food items. As we settled in at the dining room table together, I led the group in a special prayer and a toast to Angela. A couple of tears were shed, and then we proceeded to celebrate the birth of Christ, which was easier than I had anticipated. As a matter of fact, that whole day transformed from an anticipated sad one to a very joyous celebration, with all of us knowing that Angela would have wanted it to be that way.

It is very important in the grieving process to reimagine how you celebrate hot-button dates. In conjunction with my therapist, Phyllis, I have been able to rethink how I remember those days. Instead of being sad on our anniversary, for example, I now recall what a happy time our wedding was.

I am beginning to recall the joyous memories associated with these key dates instead of allowing them to cause sadness. I am learning to grasp how special it was to be together for thirty-five years, to remember the happy times and not dwell on the loss. But it takes time and focus to rethink how you remember important dates. Since Angela's death, I have learned to suppress the unhappiness of her passing. It hasn't been easy, but I have been able to recall the happy times much more often.

LESSON 10

CELEBRATE YOUR LOVED ONE'S LIFE

WHEN THE END of life comes, take the time to celebrate this special person. Create a personal tribute through writing a thoughtful memoir or obituary. In fact, the original version of this book was an extensive remembrance of Angela and our family, which I plan to share with them and our friends at a later date. How this is done perpetuates your loved one's life far beyond physical death. It allows the memory of him or her to last forever. It also produces feelings of respect and love, and calls up happy memories. For others who may have to face this event in the future, it allows them to better prepare themselves for the finality. Allow this opportunity to become a blueprint for others to copy.

In our society, the last opportunity to formally celebrate a person's life is the funeral or memorial service. It allows family and friends to communicate their loving memories through readings and words of remembrance. Your loved one becomes the focus of personal recollections, and the ritual allows all of you to begin accepting closure. This is part of the grieving process. The specifics depend on your loved one's wishes and religious affiliation. A lot of services occur in a house of worship, others in the chapel of a funeral home. Pick a venue that best fulfills the final wishes of the deceased.

After the shock of loss, accept the fact that you will come full circle in the emotions that you experienced when your loved one was still alive. Anger resurfaces almost immediately as you process the fact that what you shared in the past and your dreams for the future are now gone. You will try to affix blame to someone or something. Your faith will be tested. And that will transition into depression as you try to figure out how to live your life without your loved one.

You must grieve in your own way. There is no set schedule; everyone is different. During the first few months after Angela's death, our kids and I would ask each other how things were going and talk about it. Those questions slowly became less frequent. Family support is key in helping you and others to accept death. Moving on is a goal, but even if you never fully do so, you must learn how to live with the sadness of your loss. And don't forget to continue talking with your therapist. You need to accept that emotions will come and go, and your therapist can help you understand that they are normal.

I have found over the last year that happy memories far outweigh recollections of Angela's final illness. I believe that this is happening because of my acceptance of her death. It does not take away from the sadness of our loss, but it is allowing me to move on. I am hopeful that someday I will remember only the happy times and will be thankful for the time we had together.

A meaningful way to celebrate your loved one's life is to spend time with those who were close to him or her. Recalling the good times with others, as opposed to just yourself, will create more loving memories and remind you of the many happy times you all shared. The happier the recollection is, the more it allows you to create an inventory of memorable times, which will become greater than the stockpile of sad ones. In this way, you become happier as a person and give yourself permission to reinvent your own life. I know that this is not something you ever thought of before your loved one was struck down, but now it is reality. Your special person would never want to see you suffer through his or her demise. By celebrating that life, you will eventually be able to celebrate your own.

REFLECTIONS

DURING her two bouts with cancer and six years of treatment, Angela never complained. She was a model patient. Her treatments included radiation, chemotherapy, surgeries, scans, blood tests, experimental drugs, and physio and occupational therapies, and Angela met them all head-on. Her strength of character and strong faith allowed her to fight as long as she did. She is my hero!

I believe Angela lived so far beyond her original diagnosis not only because of her strength and faith, but also because of the love that surrounded her. She was pain-free with the brain cancer, which was a huge relief. She had an incredible care team, and numerous visits from family and friends kept her spirits high.

In my wildest dreams, I never imagined that caregiving could be such an incredible challenge, physically, mentally, and emotionally. Physically, the constant lifting and transferring, showering, bathing, and dressing and undressing someone, along with trips to the hospital and the cancer institute, can be exhausting. Mentally, being responsible for all of

Angela's medications, having to find sources of funds to pay for private caregiving at home, and being the "rock" for family members could be taxing. Emotionally, caring for a loved one who is terminally ill, wondering what you will do without that person, and always questioning whether there is more that you could do is draining. For those who do this as a career, I have nothing but sincere respect. It can be a gut-wrenching experience, and our team was exemplary.

Angela's death has left a huge void in all our lives. We had been living in Newton for fifteen years; three of our four children lived nearby for much of that time, the fourth an hour's flight away. We had many family celebrations together and will continue to do so. And we will always miss Angela.

I decided to write this book for a couple of reasons. First, as I've mentioned, my search yielded very little information for male caregivers. There were a few articles, but nothing that described the journey of a person's illness and the challenges that are inherent in caregiving. And I strongly believe that no one can fully understand this subject without experiencing it personally. Second, journaling has been shown to be an effective form of therapy in itself.

I have spent considerable time researching this subject through discussions with others who are, or who were, caregivers. If my thoughts and experiences can help someone out there who is having a difficult time in caring for a loved one, then I have completed my mission. I also hope to convince hospitals, cancer clinics, and rehab facilities everywhere to have copies of this book available to assist those who are currently, or who will become, caregivers. I completely empathize with anyone who is going through the caregiving process. My prayers and thoughts are with you all.

ABOUT THE AUTHOR

PATRICK PALMER, a former airline pilot and YMCA CEO, chairs the Angela and Patrick Palmer Research Fund for Brain Cancer, which benefits the Center for Neuro-Oncology at Dana-Farber Cancer Institute in Boston. He lives in Newton, Massachusetts.